SUDDEN DEATH

A TRUE SURVIVAL STORY

OF THROMBO EMBOLISM

MR. RICHARD P. PRENDERGAST

SUDDEN DEATH

A TRUE SURVIVAL STORY OF THROMBO EMBOLISM

by Richard P. Prendergast

CHAPTER 1

Granada

The first town you come to in the Western Alpujarros, Lanjaron is the gateway to the Granada Provence, its spa waters have been celebrated for centuries for their curative properties Overlooking the sleepy town is a ruined Moorish Castle. Legend has it that the Moorish ruler of Lanjaron threw himself from the castle tower, rather than surrender to the Catholic King Fernando.

MR. RICHARD P. PRENDERGAST

The cobbled streets are very narrow winding through the village- Chairs are outside some buildings offering rest and shelter from the siesta sun to visitors and locals alike.

Lanjaron is on the southern slopes of Spains Sierra Nevada where the air is clear and has a natural environment, mountain views and pure spring water, located on the "Old Silk Route" south to Persia .

Four thousand residents are friendly and the culture

remains thoroughly Spanish.

As you climb the mountainside you are greeted by the stark white reality of wind turbines staring at you as you drive and negotiate the dangerous unprotected corners on the cliff face.

In the village the Hotel offers parking in the shade, a fresh water swimming pool and relaxing ancient gardens.

The Hotel reception was a typical country townhouse with customary good manners and cordial welcome.

We did not need an elevator as our double ensuite room was located on the ground floor. Having deposited luggage a relaxing dip in the pool was waiting.

The weekend and holiday had begun.

It was 8 a.m on Monday when Carmela woke with her heart and head pounding. She could not breathe.!

A previous diagnosis of asthma suggested an asthmatic attack. She needed immediate medical attention. Phillip ran from the room to the reception to seek a doctors help. Paco at reception phoned the local clinic and was told that the doctor could not come. Paco brought the car to the front as Phillip grabbed an office chair with wheels and raced through the corridor, placed Carmela on the chair and dragged her to the car as she went in and out of consciousness.

Minutes later on arrival at the clinic El Doctor was unable to locate oxygen but called the ambulance crew who were based nearby. An excellent female crew member took charge and decided that a Helicopter would be needed as the road journey to

Granada would be too late.

The "Helicopteros" was also nearby and landed in a local field. The Doctor on board tried to stabilise Carmela but had great difficulty- time was critical and until she was stable they could not fly. Blood pressure was hitting the roof.

The medical air crew and ambulance crew were very professional . The Helicopter took off and headed for Hospital Universitario Virgen de las Nieves in Granada.

Granada is a city in Southern Spains Andalucia region . It has Moorish heritage going back 700 years, in the foothills of Sierra Nevada mountains. Its known for examples of medieval architecture dating to the Moorish occupation, especially the Alhambra. This sprawling hilltop fortress encompasses Royal Palaces, serene patios, and reflecting pools from the Nasrid dynasty, as well as the fountains and orchards of the Generalife gardens. The Emirs of Granada could escape the warm summers here. The Royal chapel of Granada is the ornate burial site of Catholic Kings.

In 1330 Granada was the most

densely populated city in Europe.
The coast is called Costa Tropical.

The temperature can be low
in winter dropping to just
above freezing at night.

The medical journey
had just begun.

/////////////////////////////////
////////////////////

The doctor in the helicopter assured Carmela that he would stay with her until her husband arrived and she was stable in Hospital Virgen de las Nueves (Our Lady of the Snows)

Phillip meanwhile was driving for the first time to Granada having collected passports and relevant documents that would be required by the hospital administration. He arrived at the hospital shortly after to find Carmela without a glass of water in an observation unit with thirty other patients. She was transferred to a bed in a six bed ward and at midnight taken to a nuclear / x ray department for tests. Having been returned to the ward she slept and woke throughout the night as Phillip kept vigil at her bedside. Her stomach heaved and churned during the chilly night as night nurses dozed at their station. Carmela at 7a.m, while the morning was still dark requested Phillip to return to Lanjaron to get some rest.

On his return to the hospital at 1 p.m all hell broke loose!

The hospital bed was in the centre of the ward with machines and monitors, where a team of doctors and nurses surrounding her tried to resuscitate her. Carmela needed cardioversion and was whisked away to the High Dependency Unit. Her Blood Pressure could not be lowered- she was put on Life Support.

The medical team mostly graduates from The University of Granada founded in

1531 by Emperor Charles V, could only wait- nothing more could be done.

Carmela had always insisted to her husband that should she ever be in a situation where she would be brain damaged or physically damaged she did not wish to survive. Phillip prayed for hours upon hours to Jesus and Parmahansa Yogananda(He had been a Self Realization student) to help her- the hospital chapel was visited several times but no results were forthcoming.

Clinical Reports from 40 years;

To help understand this inclusion is to give a background to patients awareness, when confronted by medical professionals understanding, of how the doctor perceives your complaint and with his training de

cides how to act and diagnose and treat or prescribe due to the limited training of the art, not the science of medicine.

Carmela attended her female General Practioner for over forty years and as a personal friend played tennis and met socially. She presented on one occassion with a panic attack and was prescribed a beta blocker . she suffered an attack while driving to work- she did not ever take a beta blocker over any period of time.

Carmela suffered breast cancer and was treated sucessfully by an eminent oncologist never to return ,Deo Gracias,

Carmela presented with Respiratory problems to a Thoracic Physician and was diagnosed with asthma and "she would have to live with it.", and to the technician in the hospital to be told she did not have a problem.! The said Professor said she had to live with the diagnosis of asthma for life and prescribed nebuliser etc. This was a mis diagnosis. Carmela never suffered from asthma and the prescribed medication is contraindicated with the official diagnosis which will be revealed later.

Carmela had been a regular swimmer, walker, cyclist. and taking a supplement of L-Arginine, Citruline, for two years previously but unfortunately did not continue for one year when tradgedy struck.

The personal trauma of one being so active and young and being subjected to a life of medication with several dietary and lifestyle changes, can be overwhelming without proper support and professional advise.

This book hopefully will show people The Light at the Start of the Tunnel. To share the experience of side effects of necessary medication and how to relieve the symptoms.

CHAPTER 2

LIFE SUPPORT

Carmela was still on "Life Support " as Phillip felt her freezing cold forehead and shoulders - her body had shut down. Any energy now was being reserved for brain function. The doctors and nurses were observing her condition continuously but there was no change. The only sounds were from the bleeps of the monitors and the suction of the breathing apparatus . She looked grey in the face and not at rest! Time passed and all sense of it was missing.

The doctors left Phillip on his own and discussed the turning off of the machines .

Phillip shouted with a startling voice as Carmela·s eyes flickered and machines bleeped. The medical team came running in and surrounded the bed as Carmela regained consciousness. She was back in the land of the living. Was there any damage done? Phillip leaned towards her and she caught his shirt with her strapped hand. He felt her feet and forehead and said - She is going to be o.k and walked down to the chapel with tears in his eyes in Thanksgiving as the medics continued with their work.

The question remained
- what caused this
Pulmonary Embolism?

A Pulmonary Embolism is the sudden blockage of a major blood vessel (artery) in the lung, usually by a blood clot (thrombus). In most cases the clots are small not deadly, but they can damage the lung, but if the clot is large and stops blood flow to the lung, it can be deadly.

A Pulmonary Embolism commonly occurs when part of the clot dislodges itself from your leg and travels up to your lungs causing a blockage.(P.E) . The blockage can cause lung damage, low oxygen levels and even death.

These embolisms affect an estimated 1 in 1000 people in the U.S. every year, 50,000-200,000 per year deaths.

.

Some symptoms can be shortness of breath and chest pain . In Carmela¨s case there was shortness of breath and heart pounding.

Across the European Union venous thrombo embolism related deaths were 12% (543,454) per annum. Incidence of P.E is estimated to be 60 to 70 per 100,000 and that of venous thrombo embolism 124 per 100,000. Silent P.E. can develop in up to 40% to 50% of patients with deep vein thrombosis (D.V.T.)

Acute P.E. ranks 3rd. among the most common types of cardiovascular disease. While clinical data indicates that most cases of P.E occur at 60 to 70 years of age, autopsy data shows the highest incidence among 70 to 80 years old. If untreated acute P.E. is associated with a significant mortality rate (as high as 30%) where as the diagnosed and treated P.E. is 8%.

Up to 10% of acute P.E. die suddenly- 2 of 3 patients succumbing to P.E. die within 2 hours after presentation.

More than half of patients experience chest pain that is sometimes difficult to distinguish from an angina of ischaemic origin. The pain experienced with P.E is usually not dull, instant, it is sharp, stinging and occasionally related to respiratory excursions. Other presentation of P.E. can include cough (approx 20% of patients) Carmela had cough also. 90% of patients present with dyspnea. (shortness of breath also known as air hunger)

Carmela remembers the thunderous clattering of the cot sides. A " Purple Cloud " enveloped the whole bed - there was no Bright Light- then there was nothing.

Carmela¨s now poor fragile body was black and blue and bruised from the necessary repeated cardioversion, the thumping and sandwiching between steel plates. Her lovely waist length hair was now in a knotted matted mass.

She was alive that was what mattered. Life is precious.

Phillip spent some time researching; he had questions to ask. He wrote down questions in English and Spanish.:

El Sindrome Troussaus ?

Estado de Hipercoagulabilidad ?

Factor V Leiden and Prothrombin G20210A. Mutation.

Factor V Leiden is a variant(mutated form) of human

Factor V (one of several substances that helps blood clot) which causes an increase in blood clotting (hypercoagulability). Due to this mutation Protein C , an anti coagulant protein which normally inhibits the pro clotting activity of Factor V, it is not able to bind normally to Factor V, leading to a Hypercoaguable State, i.e. an increased tendency for the patient to form abnormal and potentially harmful blood clots. Factor V Leiden is the most common Heredity Hyper coagulability (prone to clotting) disorder amongst ethnic Europeans.

It is named after the Dutch City Leiden where it was identified in 1994 by Prof. R Bertina under the direction of (and in the laboratory of Prof. P. Reitsma.

Leiden University is one of Europes top Universities with 13 Nobel Prize Winners. It is twinned with Oxford- the United

Kingdoms oldest University.

Phillip was in constant communication with his son who had spent some time working as a doctor in the Cardio Thoracic Department of Massachusetts General. His son had been in telephone contact with the doctors caring for Carmela.

Many samples of blood were taken from Carmela and sent for analysis to Germany.

After some time the results and cause of Carmela´s Pulmonary Embolism were confirmed.

It was the MTHFR FACTOR

(The Leiden Factor)

Now the medication challenge would follow.

CHAPTER 3

STATE OF THE ART

The medical team decided that Carmela should be transferred by ambulance to the State of the Art Health Sciences Technology Park (PTS), University Campus which houses the Faculty of Health Sciences and Faculty of Medicine, for a Greenfield Filter procedure, by the Director of the Hospital

The hospital had just opened in July 2016. This was August 2016.

The medical team wheeled Carmela through the corridors of Hospital Virgen de las Nieves to the awaiting ambulance. Phillip sat upfront as they winged their way with sirens blazing to Hospital de la Salud. The ambulance crew was never at this new hospital before.

The Director of the hospital, an interventional consultant radiologist, greeted Phillip and Carmela. Phillip walked to his office where he described the pending procedure as Carmela waited on the trolly outside the theatre . There was a risk . The consultant explained that he needed total stillness during the procedure and that usually it would take forty to forty five minutes under local anaesthetic.

The theatre had t.v screens (Sci Fi) all around with a gallery above where medical students could observe this very exact and technical procedure. The procedure took 20 minutes and the Director said Carmela was the best patient he ever had. A great success.

The main function of a vena cava filter is to prevent death from massive pulmonary emboli. Long term studies have shown that this is accomplished in 96% of cases having a standard stainless-steel Greenfield Filter.

The filter catches blood clots and stops them from moving up to the heart and lungs. This helps to prevent a pulmonary embolism. The I.V.C. filter is placed through a small incision in a vein in your groin or neck. A thin flexible tube (catheter) is inserted into the vein.

In an inferior vena cava filter placement procedure, interventional radiologists use image guidance to place the filter in the large vein in the abdomen that returns blood from the lower half of the body to the heart.

The Greenfield Filter is used to help capture clots. This type of filter is a small stainless steel device. Many filters are cone shaped with six legs that stem from the base. Each of the legs has tiny hooks on the end to help with placement and stability during the initial installation and during its use. This type of device has been used for approximately thirty years and is a well known tool in the medical world.

The Greenfield Filter promotes

the flow of blood around the device. It tapers from the base to its wider stance made by the legs so clots cannot travel any further through the vein. These are usually placed near the kidney to catch clots that may form on the legs, and travelling to the veins.

I.V.C. Filters are strategically placed to trap these clots but still allow blood to flow around them. Some are classified as permanent fixtures.

CHAPTER 4

LANJARON

Phillip had been commuting from Lanjaron to Granada each day and he would return at night. The locals new of the Emergency Helicopter and would enquire of Camela¨s well being.

As Phillip relaxed in the lobby

he noticed a Reverend nun approaching the lift dressed in a snow white habit, he spoke to her and asked her to pray for Carmela at her morning mass. She was Mother Maria, she said. The very next day was when Carmela regained consciousness. She subsequently gave Phillip a little Madonna and Child plaque to put at Carmela¨s bedside- which she still has to this day.

It was necessary for Phillip to move to a hotel in Granada after two weeks of commuting. He moved directly oposite the hospital where the new tram line had yet to be opened. In the evenings until 10 p.m. children would play on the swings and slides directly below the hospital entrance observed by their parents. Carmela had not yet seen the hospital environs.

Carmela was finally transferred to a room in the Respiratory Unit. She had lost more than 14 pounds (6.35 Kg.) . Phillip washed her matted hair using a full bottle of conditioner. She was very withdrawn and anxious about " The Purple Cloud " returning.

The regular Heparin injections caused cystitis and fortunately Phillip one evening crossed from the hotel armed with Cystopurin which relieved the problem. She was sensitive to Latex-soap also, it needed to be Intimatico . Her Obs. sheet read; Respiratorio;

Blanda Digestion

Leche Entera- Azucar,

Galletas- Descafeinado.

The little things are often forgotten-these can be major for the normal day to day comfort of the patient.

Phillip saw that Carmela was very withdrawn. She could not remember some basic happenings and slightly dragged her left foot when going to the bathroom. He decided to take her in the wheel chair down to the hospital entrance and to the Wi Fi area. As she sat there, a lovely young nurse , Anna who was part of the medical team came over to Carmela and hugged her and cried tears."you are alive you made it we were all so worried " She apologised for the chest thumping etc. and we all smiled and thanked her. We did not wish to be A-W-O-L for too long so we returned to the room. Carmela enjoyed seeing the outside of the room for the first time especially the chapel.

The Heparin Injections were painful-

Heparin is an anti coagulant (blood thinner) that prevents the formation of blood clots.

Carmela was on Bisoprolol- a medicine to treat high blood pressure (hypertension) and heart failure. Taking Bisoprolol helps prevent future heart attacks and stroke. The main side effects are feeling dizzy or sick, and headaches. Its usual to take Bisoprolol once a day in the morning. Your first dose may make you feel dizzy, so its best taken at bedtime, after that its recommended to take it in the morning.. The side effects are,; dizzy, nausea, headaches ,cold hands and feet, constipation, diarrhoea.

These are mild and transient. Carmela suffered tremendous leg pain mainly due to the after effects of the leg clots. This lasted for months. She found after a lot of switching dosage times, it was best for her to take it at eight p.m. Her dosage was 2.5 mg. daily. She had pain in all her joints. Her gums would bleed when washing her teeth. Some people tolerate this better than others.

Carmela was also prescribed Bromazepam which helped her sleep as she was so anxious and frightened that " The Purple Cloud " would return.

This was a real fear.

CHAPTER 5

DISCHARGED

Phillip and Carmela would soon be free of the hospital as she got stronger every day. The worry for Phillip was- would Carmela be able to climb the stairs etc.. Time would tell. She was now on Heperin injection into the stomach and her Bisoprolol 2.5 mg. daily and Esopremazole (Nexium) first in the morning as she does not have a gall bladder and Bromazepam at night.

The Respiratory consultant gave her the all clear. The cardiologist did E.C.G.s and required her back in the hospital after one month. She was to get Heparin injections at her local Farmacia and inject herself daily . She was free to go.

Phillip had organised a short stay in a nearby hotel (just in case) and planned to see a little part of Granada. He had not been anywhere except the hospital. Phillips son in law, offered assistance in communication if necessary, through his connections with the Order of Saint John of God who had H.Q. minutes from the hospital.

Saint John was born in Portugal in 1495. At eight years old he was placed into a Spanish family and became a shepherd in Orepesa in Spain. Twice he enlisted in the Spanish army against the French and later the Turks. After being discharged from the army, he made his way in 1538 to Granada where he made his living as a bookseller. Johns life was totally changed after hearing a sermon preached by Saint John d ·Avila in

Granada. His response was very dramatic and he became acutely aware of God's love for him and the emptiness of his life in return. His distressed appeal to God for mercy and forgiveness led him to his incarceration in The Royal Hospital for the mentally ill. As a result of this he took up the call to serve the poor and the sick , because of the mistreatment of patients he had witnessed and experienced in the hospital.

He was offered shelter in the porch of the home of Don Miguel Venegas where he brought his first patients. It was through this venture that John came to gather the support of many people including the Bishop of Granada who gave him a distinctive form of clothing, thus sowing the seeds of The Hospitaller Order of Saint John of God. Others followed in his work and his way of Life continued after his death in 1550 to this day.

In 1630 John was declared Blessed by Pope Urban V111. In 1886 he was proclaimed Patron of Hospitals and the sick and in 1930 he was further proclaimed Patron Saint of nurses and their associations by Pope Pius X1.

" For the Love of God, do good for yourselves by doing good for others ." Saint John of God-

The Granada 16 km, tram line crosses Granada from North to South and also connects the towns of Albolote and Maracena (north east) and Armilla (south east). The line serves 26 stations in total , of which just three, Mendez Nunez, Recogidas and Alcazas del Genil, are located underground in central Granada, close to the River Ganil.

Construction began in 2007. The Metro was initially planned to open in early 2012 at a cost of 500 million euro. By May 2011 when the line was 70% completed

funding ran out as a result of the Spanish economic crisis. Remaining funds were secured through a 260 million euro loan from the European Investment Bank in 2012. A further funding was required before the Metro finally opened at noon on 21st. September 2017.

The Metro serves an estimated 133,000 people who live within 500 metres of a tram station. In 2018 the actual passenger use was 10.2 million passenger journeys.

As it was August 2016, Carmela and Phillip left the Hospital Virgen de las Nieves and walked to their hotel. The broad roadway was divided by the yet to be used tramlines. The five minutes walk to the hotel has beautiful bronze statues amongst the trees and hedgerows where there is ample seating to rest . Phillip took some photographs of Carmela, now looking so much better and relaxed. The weather was beautiful and hopefully this would be the start of the convalesence.

The manager of the hotel
upgraded them to the penthouse
which had a roof terrace
where Carmela could take
the sun for a little while.

Everything was now
going to be o.k.

It was now time to return home to the Provence of Malaga . The arrival home would be quiet as nobody in the little community was aware of Carmela¨ s near death experience.

Malaga is a port city in
Southern Spains Costa del Sol
with yellow sandy beaches.
Over the modern skyline

are the citys two massive hilltop citadels.(The Alcazaba and ruined Gibralfaro,) . The citys soaring Renaissance Cathedral is nicknamed La Manquita (one armed lady) because one of the towers was left unbuilt for some unknown reason.

Of course there is The Museo Picasso in Malaga- where Pablo Picasso was born in 1881. The museum opened in 2003 in the Buenavista Palace and has 285 works donated by members of the Picasso family.

Malaga is one of the oldest cities in the world and has 3000 years of history.

The Phoenicians first colonized the city in 1000 B.C. and named it Malaka. from the Phoenician word "to salt" as The Gualdalhorce River was the fish salting centre. The area was rich in metals like silver and copper. The Greeks also came and settled in the area in the 6th century . The Greek rule ended in 550 B.C. when the Carthaginians attacked and took control. The Romans conquered the city in the 3rd century and named it Flavia Malacita. The port was used to export oil, raisins, wine and salted fish and meat. The Roman amphitheatre was then constructed.

Following the Moorish conquest 714-716 and the rise and fall of various Muslim dynasties, the city eventually fell under the control of the Nasrids (.Granada) . Enjoying great prosperity due to the development of the textile industry.

It took nearly 100 years before the Christians managed to conquer the city, doing so in 1487. In the 19 th. century two wealthy families Heredia (iron & steel) and the Larios (textiles) based their factories in Malaga.

The 20th century brought
very difficult times-natural disasters, earthquakes,plagues, and failed harvests.

The political instability during

this period culminated with the Spanish Civil War. Malaga fell to Pro Franco forces on 8th February 1937. Over 120,000 people many civilians were forced to abandon their city by foot along the old Almeria road (N340) attempting to walk 200 km.They were under constant fire from Franco¨ s troops (backed by Italian and German aerial and marine forces) from the sea, the air, and on land. Many thousands of innocent civilians lost their lives enroute and afterwards. This was called " The Caravan of Death". The Desbanda is commemorated every year in Torre del Mar on 7th. February.

The 1950 s saw the beginning of a new era in Malaga and Costa del Sol. Tourism was beginning to take hold.

Visiting Malaga today is like walking around an open air Museum with Christian, Moorish, Roman , and Phoenician influences.

Carmela continued with her Heparin Injections and her treatment together with Bisoprolol 2.5 mg and Bromazepam 1.5 mg. She still suffered the side effects of severe joint pain and the cystitis was also evident. She returned to Granada for her appointments with the Vascular surgeon and her Cardiologist. She was prescribed Sintrom (acenocoumarol) an anti coagulant to be taken orally similar to Warfarin instead of the Heparin Injection together with her Bisoprolol, Paracetamol etc. It would be necessary to visit her local hospital or clinic regularly to assess her progress i.e. to measure her I.N.R..

The Independent Normalized Ratio (I.N.R.) is the standardized number from the laboratory. In healthy people a result of 1 up to 1.5 is considered normal. An I.N.R. of 2 to 3. is generally an effective therapeutic range for people taking Coumadrin or Acenocoumarol for disorders such as atrial fibrillation or a blood clot in the leg or lung. If the I.N.R. is too low, blood clots will not be prevented, but if the I.N.R. is too high, there is an

increased risk of bleeding. A low I.N.R means your blood is not thin enough or coagulates too easily and you risk bleeding.

It was necessary for Carmela to visit Hospital Costa del Sol in Marbella to have her blood checked on a regular basis. Early in the morning before the worker traffic heading South to Cadiz, Jerez, and Marbella , Phillip would drive her to the hospital .

Hospital Costa del Sol is on the coast road 7 km. east of Marbella. Its one of the best equipped hospitals in Spain. Inaugurated in 1993 and run as an independent company on behalf of S.A.S. Andalucian Health Authority.. It has 400 beds. Sometimes voluntary interpreters are available to help other nationalities communicate with the medical staff, 15% of patients being non Spanish speakers- this is considered a necessity for the smooth running of the hospital. In summer the average number of emergencies increases from 140 to 355 a day.

In 2008 an extension was started that will on completion offer another 150 beds and a number of additional specialities. Currently only part of the extension to be opened is the underground car park.

Having queued for some time with many others for the blood sample to be taken , it was necessary to wait about two hours for the result of the I.N.R. to be logged in the computer and for the next procedure to be announced. If the medication was to be adjusted up or down it would then be necessary to return in a few days for further samples to be taken. This journey to the hospital continued for several weeks.

Some foods were limited while on anticoagulants. Foods rich in Vitamin K were to be avoided as this is part of the coagulating factor while on Warfarin or Sintrom.

Vitamin K rich;

Kale, Spinach, Brussels Sprouts, Parsley, Collard Greens. Mustard Greens, Red Cabbage, Green lettuce. Avoid Green Tea as it contains Vitamin K, Grapefruit, Cranberry Juice, and Alcohol..

However low in Vitamin K are ;

Sweetcorn, Onions, Squash, Eggplant, Tomatoes, Mushrooms,

Sweet Potatoes, Cucumber (raw), Artichoke, Strawberries, Apples, Peaches, Watermelon, Pineapple and Bananas.

Phillip discovered that a Coagucheck System could be purchased to monitor the I.N.R. levels at home and reduce the number of hospital visits to periodic ones-

A Coagucheck XS system is a convenient , portable and user friendly instrument for monitoring anticoagulent therapy. It determines the I.N.R.value from a drop of capillary whole blood and saves the patient endless hours travel time to hospital or clinic. The patient can readily monitor their I.N.R. and contact their own medical practioner for dosage adjustment as necessary.

CHAPTER 6

MTHFR

Carmela reflects on how the hidden genetic dormant MTHFR (Leidin Factor) manifested itself , as she was active all her life - playing tennis, swimming, going to the gym and even training and running a mini marathon.

She remembers that in 2013 at 4 a.m she was short of breath, her lips were swollen and she needed immediate medical attention. It appeared as if she had an allergic reaction to something she had eaten a few hours before. She had eaten a chinese take away.

Phillip drove her to an emergency clinic as she could not breathe. the doctor gave her an injection and sent her by ambulance to St. Vincents Hospital Dublin , Accident & Emergency Department. She was put on a drip and then left in observation for a few hours.

Carmela was released from hospital and given a prescription for an Epi Pen - Epinephrine Auto Injector (a disposable pre filled automatic medical device for injecting a measured dose. Epinephrine, a chemical that narrows blood vessels and opens airways in the lungs. These effects can reverse severe low blood pressure, wheezing and other symptoms of an allergic reaction. Epinephrine increases blood pressure and can trigger heart arrhythmias, strokes and heart attacks.

Carmela was discharged on the same day. She returned home

and a few days later visited her General Practioner who made an appointment with an allergy specialist in Dublin. The diagnosis after the" patient in hospital Allergy Challenge", Carmela was only allergic to mould - like 95% of the rest of the population.

Carmela attended her General Practioner who prescribed an inhaler for her (Salbutamol) and referred her to a Consultant Respiratory Physician.

Carmela had a series of laboratory Pulmonary Function Tests conducted by a specialist nurse. The result was no asthma and no need for inhalers. Her lung function was perfect.

Carmela attended the appointment and was told she had asthma and the Prof. said " you will have to live with it ".

CHAPTER 7

CERTIFICATE OF FITNESS

Carmela got a Certificate of Fitness from the Hospital to fly home to Ireland.

She spent a little while relaxing with family in Kilkenny.

Kilkenny is a medieval City in the South East of Ireland.

Kilkenny Castle was built in 1195 by Norman occupiers.

The City has deep religious roots and many well preserved churches and monasteries including the imposing Saint Canices Cathedral and The Black Abbey- Dominican Priory both from the 13th Century. Its also a craft hub with pottery, paintings and jewellery.

It is situated on both banks of the River Nore.

The City of Kilkenny is often referred to as "The Marble City ". The footpaths of the city streets were paved with limestone flagstones, which when wet , glistened. A very dark grey limestone was quarried just outside the City in a place known as the Black Quarry due to the colour of the final product.

Carmela while there, dined in a restaurant and had severe consequences. She got palpitations and thought this might be due to M.S.G. " Monosodium Glutamate "- food flavour enhanser, as it happened previously ! A visit to her doctor revealed elevated blood pressure and an ambulance would be necessary. An E.C.G was done also.

Carmela was now in Accident & Emergency at Wexford General Hospital. The same procedure again trying to reduce her blood pressure. The following morning they decided to transfer Carmela back to St. Vincents Hospital in Dublin by special cardiac ambulance and team. Wexford did not have sufficient cardiac facilities to deal with her situation..

Carmela had an Angiogram done (an x ray procedure that can be both diagnostic and therapeutic.) It is considered the gold standard for evaluating blockages in the arterial system. An angiogram detects blockages using x-rays taken during the injection of a contrast

agent (iodine dye). It didnt reveal any blockages in her heart. She returned home with an appointment to see the Professor. This was a very anxious time

The Professors Registrar decided to put Carmela on a monitor day and night for a week. This would tell how her medication was acting.

The Registrar thought that Carmela was suffering considerably and should consider having a heart ablation as she was too young to have to cope with the hardship.

Cardiac ablation is a procedure using radiofrequency energy (similar to microwave heat) to scar or destroy tissue in your heart thats allowing incorrect electrical signals to cause an abnormal heart rhythm. Diagnostic catheters are threaded through blood vessels to your heart where they are used to map your hearts electrical signals .

The burns irritate the heart, and as they heal (expand), over days to weeks, the irregular rhythm can resolve. This is why we have what is called a waiting period (6- 8 weeks) after the procedure., before a success or not, is declared.

When the procedure is repeated in patients who still have atrial fibrillation after the first procedure, the overall success rate is approximately 85% to 90%. Persistant atrial fibrillation can be eliminated in approx. 50% of patients with a single procedure.

Once the tissue is destroyed, the abnormal electrical signals that created the arrhythmia can no longer be sent to the rest of the heart. Most people do not feel pain during the procedure which is done under local anaesthesia. Mild discomfort may be felt.

The heart has its own electrical conduction system. It sends signals throughout the upper chamber (atria) and lower chambers (ventricles) of the heart to make it beat in a regular co-ordinated rhythm. The conduction consists of two nodes that contain conduction cells and special pathways that transmit the impulse.

A normal heartbeat begins when an electrical impulse is fired from the sinus node (also called sino atrial node or SA node) in the right atrium.

The sinus node is responsible for setting the rate and rhythm of the heart and is therefore referred to as the Pacemaker.

The electrical impulse fired from the SA node spreads throughout the atria, causing them to contract and squeeze blood into the ventricles.

The electrical impulse then reaches the atrio ventricular node (AV node) which acts as a gateway, slowing and regulating the impulses travelling between the atria and the ventricles. As an impulse travels down the pathway into the ventricles the heart contracts and pumps blood around the body. The cycle then begins again.

A normal adults heart beats in a regular pattern 60 to 100 times a minute. This is called sinus rhythm.

Sometimes if the conduction pathway is damaged,blocked or an extra pathway exists, the heart rhythm

changes. The heart may beat too quickly (tachycardia) or too slowly (bradycardia) or irregularly. This may affect the hearts ability to pump blood around the body. These abnormal heartbeats are known as arrhythmias. Arrhythmias can occur in the atria and in the ventricals.

Carmela would now have to consider this procedure.

The MTHFR (Methylene Tetra Hydro Folate Reductase) is a gene. Genes are the basic units of heredity passed down from father and mother.

Everyone has two MTHFR genes one from the father and the other from the mother.. Mutations or variants can occur in one or both genes. There are different types of variants -C677T & A1298C. The MTHFR gene helps your body break down a substance called homocysteine, an amino acid, a chemical in your body to make proteins. Normally folic acid and other B vitamins break down homocysteine and change it into other substances your body needs. There should then be very little homocysteine left in the blood stream. If you have a MTHFR mutation your MTHFR gene may not work correctly. This may cause too much homocysteine to

build up in the blood,
leading to various health

problems including;

Homocystinurea- a disorder that affects the eyes, joints and cognitive abilities. It usually starts in early childhood.

An increased risk of heart disease,stroke,high blood pressure and blood clots.

In addition women with MTHFR mutation can have a higher risk of having a baby with Spina Bifida.

You can reduce homocysteine levels by taking Folic acid or other B vitamin supplements added to your diet, enough to keep homocysteine levels within range .

An individual can function properly even with a lower than normal level of the enzyme as long as there is enough to keep homocysteine levels within a healthy range.

Having a single copy of the variants does not decrease the activity of the enzyme. Mutations occur in over 25% of Hispanic descent and 10% to 15% of European descent.

MR. RICHARD P. PRENDERGAST

For the majority of people with a common MTHFR variant, they will not have any symptoms and the overall health risks associated with a common variant are so small (or non existant for many) that they would not need any course of treatment. Simply put, having an MTHFR variant doesnt mean you need any treatment.

If your symptomless and curious rather than going down the genetic testing route- get a blood test to check your homocysteine levels, which is a real indicator of

potential health issues.

Its less expensive and it can tell you, if anything is actually wrong clinically.

Clinically significant MTHFR gene mutations would be indicated by abnormally high homocysteine levels.

If high, homocysteine treatment is simple with Folate supplements which help your body to bypass the need for MTHFR enzyme- regular folate works , B6 AND B12 for some people on your doctors advice.

CHAPTER 8

LUNG FUNCTION

In June 2015 Carmela had an episode of not being able to walk and she had diminished lung function. She visited the General Practioners office and he treated her - gave her oxygen and an injection and said that she had a severe lung infection . Having treated her every week for six weeks with repeated injections , her condition was not improving.

She was admitted to hospital with Bilateral Pneumonia and treated as an in patient for 15 days. There was fluid on her two lungs and the doctors decided to remove it the next morning. An x-ray was ordered prior to the procedure to find that overnight the fluid had gone! Where did it go ?

Carmela was discharged after the 15 days with strong antibiotics to be taken orally for two months because the doctor said there was a small shadow left in the right lung which would disappear with the medication. The question must be asked " was this a clot " ?

Carmela has initially been treated for Asthma, and prescribed ;

Salbutamol; A medication that opens up the medium and large airways in the lungs. Its used to treat asthma, including exercise induced asthma attacks. Broncho constriction and chronic obstructive pulmonary disease.

Serotide; This is indicated for the symptomatic treatment of patients with COPD (Chronic

Obstructive Pulmonary Disease) and a history of repeated exacerbations which have significant symptoms.

Carmela had also had a nebuliser for use in an emergency situation.

This of course would exacerbate her condition especially when she had ultimately been diagnosed with

The Leidin Factor (MTHFR) and had been prescribed the necessary medication for this condition. Some of the existing medication that had been prescribed previously would be contraindicated now with this proper diagnosis. Carmela had been through so much suffer

ing due to the missed diagnosis initially, when she presented with a so called allergy , and having been treated for asthma when in fact she never had asthma.!!!

On the 17th 0f August 2016 Carmela had been diagnosed with ;

Cardiorespiratory Arrest, Secondary Bilateral Pulmonary Embolism, Deep Vein

Thrombus(two legs) DVT- with need for Cava filter.

In Critical care she was administered ;

Amiodarone- this is used to treat certain types of serious (possibly fatal) irregular heartbeat (such as persistent ventricular fibrillation - tachycardia) It is used to restore normal heart function and to maintain a regular steady heartbeat. Its known as a anti arrhythmic drug. It also causes blood vessels to dilate. The result can be a drop in Blood Pressure. She was also administered Tinzaparina - an anti thrombotic drug in the

Heparin Group for prevention of D.V.T and Pulmonary Embolism, (P.E)

Carmela was prescribed Bisoprolol 2.5 mg . This is a beta blocker used to treat Blood Pressure and hypertension and heart failure. to prevent future heart attacks and

stroke. This medication relaxes blood vessels and slows heart rate and decreases Blood Pressure.

Bromazepam as an anxiolytic to treat panic attacks was also given at night.

Esopremazole also, in the morning to help tolerate all the medication.

Carmela was back at the hospital in Dublin again.

Dublin is the capital of the Republic of Ireland and is on the east coast at the mouth of the River Liffey. Its historic buildings include- Dublin Castle, dating from the 13th century and the imposing Saint Patricks Cathedral , founded in 1191.

City Parks include landscaped Saint Stephens Green and the Phoenix Park.

Aras an Uachtarain "House of the President ", formerly the Viceroy Lodge, is the official residence and work place of the President of Ireland. It is located off Chesterfield Avenue in the Phoenix Park. The building has 95 rooms and was designed by Nathaniel Clements and completed in 1751.

Dublin Zoo is also in the Phoenix Park, established and designed in 1830 by Decimus Burton and its role is conservation, study, and education.

In 1838 to celebrate Queen Victoria¨s coronation, Dublin Zoo held an" open day" and

20,000 people visited there.

Leinster House is the seat of rhe Oireachtas, the Parliament of Ireland. Originally the Ducal Palace of the Duke of Leinster. When the Earl became the First Duke of Leinster in 1766, the Dublin residence was renamed Leinster House.

The Mansion House in Dawson Street Dublin, has been the official residence of the Lord Mayor of Dublin since 1715, and was also the meeting place of Dail Eireann

(Parliament) from 1919 to 1922. It was built in 1710 by

the merchant and property developer Joshua Dawson , whose name is commemorated in Dawson Street.

Christ Church Cathedral- The Cathedral of The Holy Trinity (Church of Ireland) is another of the many historic buildings in the city.

A visit to Dublin is not complete without a visit to Guinness Brewery.

Arthur Guinness started brewing ale in 1759 at Saint James Gate, on 31 st. December. He signed a 9,000 year lease at 45 pounds per annum for the unused brewery.

Ten years later 1769 Guinness first exported his ale - He shipped six and a half million Barrels to

Great Britain.

Following another consultation at St. Vincents Hospital it was decided to change Carmela¨s medication- to stop Bisoprolol and change to Sotalol:

Sotalol is a medication used

to treat and prevent abnormal heart rhythms. It is only recommended in those with significant abnormal heart rhythms due to potentially serious side effects. Evidence does not support a decreased risk of death with long term use.

For the first three days taking Sotalol you need to be in a facility where your heart can be monitored as it can cause irregular heart beats.

Sotalol is an antiarrhythmic - it works on the heart muscle to improve the heart rhythm.

Sintrom was changed to a new anticoagulant Apixaban. There was no need to measure I.N.R. (International Normalized Ratio)- The I.N.R. is calculated using the results of the Prothrombin time (PT) test, discussed earlier in this book.

CHAPTER 9

NATURAL CURES

The advances made in medical technology, medicine and nursing training have been very significant in the last few years. There is a great emphasis on new drug development from the major Pharmaceutical companies while many natural cures are overlooked.

Does your blood flow freely through your arteries and veins or is it viscous and sticky (hyperviscosity ?) Studies confirm that sticky blood is a huge factor for strokes and heart attacks and other cardiovascular problems because sticky blood is harder for your heart to pump around your body and is far more likely to clot. Mainstream medicine turns to drugs (anticoagulants),

when you present with blood problems. We are very grateful to have these medications.

IF YOU HAVENT BEEN DIAGNOSED AT RISK --
from heart attack or stroke conditions, What can you do?

Donate blood- If you donate blood regularly it helps thin your blood reducing damage to your blood vessels and possibly preventing blockages. It was suggested that this could be a reason for some menstruating women not having heart attacks and stroke..

Diet ; Add garlic to your diet (not if you are on blood thinners) to help prevent blood platelets from sticking together, reducing the risk of clots.

Allicin is the active part in garlic, and preferably eaten raw, as allicin is destroyed at high temperatures. Add towards the end of cooking.

Vitamin E. (d - alpha - tocopherol). People with the lowest Vitamin E levels had the highest risk of heart disease and stroke.

Fish oil: Omega-3 reduces inflammation, lowers cholesterol. If you are taking anticoagulants you must talk to your doctor before taking Omega-3 or any supplements.

Drink plenty of water- staying hydrated is essential and often overlooked especially if you have a history of heart disease. You can make your blood less sticky by drinking plenty of water.

Many people take Aspirin , it can come with serious potential side effects. The drug can lead to gastrointestinal bleeding for some people and for some it can do more harm than thought before.

Aspirin is a synthesised version of the active component of an extract found in the bark of the Willow tree.

Instead of aspirin, a white willow supplement can give you the benefits. without the side effects.

Even though the British and Irish have similar intake of saturated fats as the French, heart disease is lower in France. It may be due to their consumption of red

wine. Red wine is rich in OPC ¨s (oligomeric procyanidins). The quality of the wine makes a difference. Wine without preservatives (sulphites) is better. Limited of course to one or two glasses per day ! Resveratrol supplement has the same effect but often wine is preferred ! Hawthorn is also high in OPC¨s and has been used medically for years.

Cholesterol ; Cholesterol levels need to be monitored.

Cholesterol lowering foods are ;

Garlic, onions ,Oat bran, carrots, etc.

Drugs are seldom necessary as there are several alternatives to lowering cholesterol; vitamins, minerals, and botanicals. e.g Vitamin C. Calcium , Magnesium, Vitamin E. L-Carnithine, Lecithin, Beta - sitosterol, these raise

HDL good cholesterol also Turmeric , curcumin, reishi mushrooms , fenu greek.

` ` `

Magnesium has not been recognised for some time as being a very valuable part of your diet. It helps to promote strong bones, a good nights sleep , and most importantly it can be the key factor in protecting your heart and even preventing a heart attack. Magnesium has not been appreciated in its fight against inflammation, and inflammation is the reason why your bodies organs break down including your cardiovascular system. When the lining of your arteries becomes in

flamed , your body produces C-reactive protein, nuclear factor kappa B, and cytokines, and puts platelets on the injured cells in the process called Thrombosis. Using cholesterol and other substances , your body tries to heal the wound. This area (atheroma) collects calcium and fibrous tissue which hardens into plaque and obstructs the artery- that is when a condition of atherosclerosis occurs.

Hardened arteries lead to high blood pressure and atherosclerotic cardiovascular disease . (ASCVD).

It is unlikely that you will go through this if you have sufficient Magnesium . Dietary magnesium can prevent arterial clot formation and therefore prevent ASCVD. Magnesium can help your good cholesterol and keep your

blood pressure from going high .

The heart is a muscle and it needs to be relaxed. If you have too much calcium in the cells it can result in muscle contraction. Magnesium is your body¨s natural calcium blocker.

When magnesium moves from inside your body cells, through the cell membrane to outside the cell, it blocks calcium from entering the cells. There is then less pro

duction of the two main hormones that contribute to high blood pressure- aldosterone and angiotensin and the result is lowered blood pressure.

Magnesium lowers L.D.L (bad) cholesterol and increases HDL (good cholesterol).

Magnesium can work in the same way as statins without the side effects. It inhibits HMG-

Co A., the enzyme that makes cholesterol in your body.

If you have atherosclerotic cardiovascular disease studies show that magnesium can prevent it from worsening and may help to improve the condition.

As your risk of stroke increases with atrial fibrillation, a dangerous complication of cardiovascular surgery that can be lessened by magnesium before surgery. A study shows that only 2% of patients treated with IV magnesium sulphate before cardiac bypass surgery, experienced the irregular heart rate associated with atrial fibrillation towards 21% of the untreated group.

A magnesium rich diet includes :

Spinach, and other dark green leafy vegetables. (not while taking coumadrin),

Bananas, nuts and seeds,

Fish, Avocado, and even - Dark chocolate.

CHAPTER 10

HOMOCYSTEINE

When Carmela presented in hospital in 2015 and she was told she had asthma- why were her homocysteine levels not checked or discussed ?

Homocysteine levels can become dangerously high.

Homocysteine is made when you consume food with animal and vegetable protein with the amino acid methionine- this breaks down the homocysteine which converts back to amino acids, with the presence of Vitamin B 6. This process keeps homocysteine levels normal. However if you are low in Vitamin B 6 and have a high intake of methionine a problem can arise.

With modern farming and food processing we do not get sufficient Vitamins B 6, B 12, and Folic Acid, so it may be necessary to supplement with multivitamins.

Carmela two years prior to 2015 had been supplementing with L-Citruline,L-Arginine. (Pro- Argi 9) this helps with the production of Nitric Oxide, but alas stopped. This may have helped or delayed the onset of her Pulmonary Embolism until August 2016.

The Nobel Prize in 1998 in Physiology and Medicine was awarded to North American Drs. Robert F. Furchgott, Louis J. Ignarro and Ferid Murad for their discoveries in relation to Nitric Oxide as a signalling molecule in the cardiovascular system. It was felt that Dr. Salvador Moncada should have been included for his work.

**Nitric Oxide is released by endothelial cells.

Nitric Oxide helps to ;

Prevent high blood pressure, clots and plaque build up.

Lowers C - Reactive Protein (C. R. P.) and reduces triglyceride levels.

Nitric Oxide helps to reduce the risk of heart attacks and stroke.

The endothelial cells line all blood vessels and produce Nitric Oxide, but as you get older less is produced. It helps smooth muscle relax and dilates arteries reducing the peripheral resistance . This is called vasodilation. If the arteries are like concrete pipes the colateral circulation must be helped.

With the help of dilating the arteries the blood flow increases throughout the body including the extremities.

Men with Erectile Disfunction (E. D.) may find benefit from increased Nitric Oxide levels.

When you are deficient in N.O. your arteries can not relax and remain narrow and inflexible, allowing plaque to manifest itself. This increases cardiac risk ! Chronic inflammation occurs in your arteries and oxidative stress begins. Inflammation and oxidation to-gether help plaque burst open and toxins are released.

which can trigger blood clots in your arteries. Nitric Oxide levels can prevent this.

Triglyceride levels fall, and C.R.P (C- Reactive Protein)

Systolic and Diastolic Blood Pressure are normalised.

Vitamin C promotes the availability of Nitric Oxide and strengthens your arteries and is a potent antioxidant. Vitamin B12 plays a very important role in your cardiovascular system- you can not make red blood cells without it.

L- Citrulline is directly involved in N.O. production and shown to reverse the progression of atheroslerosis. L-Citrulline converts to L- Arginine and is needed in combination as L- Arginine on its own is excreted very quickly .

The medical profession is often divided about treatments .

" Doctors differ and patients die ", This is a very old saying.

Saturated fats and cholesterol have received very bad press in the last few decades so most people think that they should avoid them. New research reveals that there is no actual observed connection between saturated fats and coronary heart disease. A study at Cambridge University of 600,000 people- 72 studies and

18 countries found no link between saturated fats and heart disease. The complete opposite of what we knew heretofore.

For years the mainstream media has demonized foods like eggs and meats, they claimed that they were the cause of all sorts of disease. This was wrong as the latest science has shown.

Eggs while long known to be a nutritious food, have also been demonized due to their high cholesterol content. We have been told this for years that foods containing cholesterol may lead to heart disease and can raise the risk of type 2 diabetes. Now however nutritious sources of cholesterol and saturated fats are not bad for us and new research has found that eggs may actually lower type 2 diabetes risk- University of Finland, published in America Journal of Clinical Nutrition. The study over 20 years with 2,400 men aged between 42 years and 60 years- Researchers linked eating an average of four eggs per week with a 37% lower risk

of receiving a type 2 diabetes diagnosis as compared to men who ate an average of one egg per week. The researchers associated eating eggs with lower blood sugar levels. Higher egg consumption was associated with a lower risk of type 2 diabetes in middle aged men.

One component of food such as cholesterol does not characterize the nutritional merit of the said food.

Eggs are a whole food from Mother Nature and their nutritional make up is complex which may explain their effect on lowering blood sugar.

Eggs and saturated fats are not the enemy.!

` ` ` ` ` ` ` ` ` ` ` ` ` ` ` ` ` ` ` ` ` ` ` ` ` ` ` `
` ` ` ` ` ` ` ` ` ` ` ` ` `

Another hospital consultation in 2018 ;

Carmela continued to have pain in two legs and fatigue. She continued to exercise and push herself to cycle and walk early in the morning. She suffered from depression due to the medication but did not succumb to any medication. She always had great determination in beating this ongoing challenge.

Her medication was changed to include Dromaderone (Multaq 400 mg) together with her Apixaban (Eliquis) the anticoagulant instead of Sintrom.

Dronaderone is used to treat people who currently have a normal heart rhythm but have had atrial fibrillation in the past. The drug reduces the risk of further hospitalization. The dosage is 400 mg. twice daily . Dronaderone is related to Amiodarone which is the drug of choice in hospital admissions to stabilise atrial fibrillation.

Initially Carmela has to take medication at prescribed times of the day but this changed due to side effects experienced. People will differ. She took 400mg. at 11 a.m - this was too late in the day as you may experience gastric upset and may need to use the bathroom. So over time it was shown that for her it was best to take /

Dronaderone at 8.a.m during breakfast. This made a great difference in tolerating the medication. Similarly in the evening to take the medication during dinner. It is necessary to adjust your times to suit your own lifestyle but must be taken with meals.

Each month Carmela experienced two days of lethargy and leg pain but when these past, all was o.k. There can be no missing of any medication at any time, so it is ideal to have tablets in plastic dated containers, which are readily available.

It is of great importance to push oneself to get outdoors and walk, exercise, cycle, and not let these conditions get the better of you and live a full life.

CHAPTER 11

RELAXATION

Carmela had an appointment with her Cardiologist in Spain to review her present condition and have ECG and bloods done.

She is very afraid of flying since her episode so Phillip decided to treat her to a little break and drive via United Kingdom to spend a few days in Wales,; and see relations there, and then journey on from Plymouth to Santander .

The best route is The ancient Roman Silver Route "Ruta de la Plata ", from Palencia Spain to Seville.

During the reigns of Emperor Trajan and Hadrian a route that linked the Cantabrian coast with the lands of the south of Hispania, a grand access route was created in the west of the peninsula .

Goods, troops, traders and travellers moved along this trail, which favoured the spreading of Roman culture, its language and way of life, at the same time as facilitating the control of the territory that the administration of the Roman Empire required.

The trail continued to be used over the centuries, both by Arabs as well as Christians during the middle ages, and went on to play an important role in the communications network of the Iberian Peninsula.

The Romans built several thousand kilometres of roads, feats of engineering- of bridges which 2,000 years later remain as monuments, at the same time as fulfilling their original function.

Carmela and Phillip stopped over in Palencia before their onward journey to Salamanca on the Silver Route.

Salamanca is considered to be one of the safest cities in Spain. Violent crime is for the most part unheard of. The University of Salamanca Founded in the 1100 s is the 3rd. oldest in Europe.

It was necessary for Carmela to have a period of relaxation as she had been through so much pain . Her pain threshold is very high. It appears that women are better able to cope with pain than men.

Her son and daughter-in-law had booked a country cottage in Saint Ives , Cornwall for her, so she could unwind and have total relaxation for a week. She had never been to this part of the United Kingdom. This was a special treat as she could meet her grand children whom she had not seen for a considerable time.

On arrival at the cottage, a beautiful picturesque farm, freshly baked scones with melted butter and strawberry jam and Devon cream awaited.

She would later visit the famous Tin Mines.

Historically, tin and copper as well as a few other metals, (arsenic, silver, and zinc) have been mined in

Cornwall and Devon. As of 2007 there are no active metalliferous mines remaining. Tin deposits still exist.

The Cornwall and West Devon Mining landscape is a World Heritage site and certainly should not be missed. Cambourne School of Mines was founded in 1888 and developed as the only specialist hard rock education establishment in the U.K. It continues to teach mining as well as engineering geology. It is part of the University of Leicester. Graduates of Cambourne are to be found working in the mining industry all over the world. The Royal Geological Society of Cornwall was founded in 1814 and is the 2nd. oldest geological society in the world.

CHAPTER 12

CACERES

The journey continued on to Caceres a city in western Spain founded by the ancient Romans. Caceres , a medieval hidden gem of a destination, is one of Spains most underrated cities about four hours drive from Malaga.

Its architecture is of Roman, Islamic, Northern Gothic and Italian Renaissance styles . Of the 30 towers from the Muslim Period the "Torre de Bujaco" is the most famous.

Seville was the second last stop, the capital of southern Spains Andalucia region. World famous for its culture,

monuments, traditions and artistic heritage. Seville is the birthplace of " Flamenco "

The heart of Seville is Santa Cruz, one of the most beautiful barrios (neighbourhoods) in Spain. Next stop Malaga and journeys end.

Carmela had her E.C.G done and her bloods checked and all was perfect , the cardiologist was pleased. One more change of medications the cardiologist ordered, that was a change from Apixaban (Eliquis) to Edoxaban (Lixiana).

Carmela had come a long way. There was now a " Light at the End of the Tunnel ".

Despite that the medication causes weight gain and the two bad days in the month remain , life is well worth living.

Carmela never cycled a bicycle
since she was a child and
that was a " three wheeler",
she fell from that one.!!

Now she has progressed
to a mountain bike having
traded in her " Mary Poppins
" city bike with the basket
and flowers in front.-

Carmela is very grateful to God
for sparing her life and for giving
her a second " bite of the cherry ".

She is also thankful to all the
people in all the clinics and hos-

pitals that she attended and especially to the ambulance and helicopter medical crews that helped save her life.

" Go mbeirimid beo ar an am seo aris . " (IRISH)

" May we all be alive at this time (again) next year.
" ------   Carmela

Carmela.

Acknowledgements

The ambulance crew in Lanjaron.

The doctor and Helicopter crew

All the medical and nursing staff at Hospital Universitario Virgen de las Nieves.

The Cardiology & Respiratory Teams.

The Consultant at Hospital PTS Parque Tecnologico de la Salud.

The reception staff at Hotel Andalucia Lanjaron, and Reverend Mother.

Family and friends for their continuing support.

To the Medical & Pharmaceutical Researchers

To my husband who made everything possible to get me through this journey, with meditation and prayers.

THANK YOU.

REVIEW

Its very important to consult your medical adviser.

Readers should consult appropriate health professionals on any matter relating to their health and well being.

The contents herein are for information only and may not be construed as instruction or medical advice.

Take medication as prescribed - during meals as necessary, vary times dependant on side effects.

Its good to practice meditation and to be in the right frame of mind when dealing with your pain.

Rest is essential when your body tells you to.

Get walking when ever your schedule allows.

Watch your diet and yet treat yourself with rewards when you deserve them.

Life and Shade by turn but Love Always.

This book is a true account of a very long journey of survival through many medical diagnoses and treatments.

The information may help people to seek medical attention sooner.

COPYRIGHT 2019. ALL RIGHTS RESERVED. NO PART OF THIS BOOK MAY BE REPRODUCED BY ANY MEANS OR

for any reason without consent.

All material in this publication is for information only and not to be construed as advice or instruction.

All rights reserved.

No action should be taken based on the contents heirin instead readers should consult appropriate health professionals in relation to their own health.

The publisher is not responsible for any errors or

omissions.

www.ingramcontent.com/pod-product-compliance
Lightning Source LLC
Chambersburg PA
CBHW021418210526
45463CB00001B/428